First published 2020 by Picador
an imprint of Pan Macmillan
The Smithson, 6 Briset Street, London EC1M 5NR
Associated companies throughout the world
www.panmacmillan.com

ISBN 978-1-5290-3403-5

Copyright © Adam Kay 2020

The right of Adam Kay to be identified as the author
of this work has been asserted by him in accordance with
the Copyright, Designs and Patents Act 1988.

Pan Macmillan does not have any control over, or any responsibility for,
any author or third-party websites referred to in or on this book.

9 8 7 6 5 4 3 2

A CIP catalogue record for this book is available from the British Library.

Printed and bound by CPI Group (UK) Ltd, Croydon, CR0 4YY

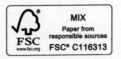

Visit www.picador.com to read more about all our books
and to buy them. You will also find features, author interviews and
news of any author events, and you can sign up for e-newsletters
so that you're always first to hear about our new releases.

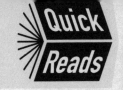
Quick Reads
This is Going to Hurt

Adam Kay

Specially rewritten for ease of
reading by Francesca Main

PICADOR

This is an edited extract from *This is Going to Hurt: Secret Diaries of a Junior Doctor*, rewritten for ease of reading. Everything you will read is true but names, dates and some details have been changed to protect the people in the book.

In 2010, I left my job as a junior doctor. My parents will probably never forgive me.

Last year, I was sent a letter that said I would never be able to work as a doctor again. It wasn't a big shock, as I had not set foot in a hospital for so long. But I still found it sad that this part of my life had come to an end.

It was good news for my spare room at least. I cleared out box after box of papers, and the only things that I saved were my old diaries. As I read through the stories – some funny, some sad, some painful – I remembered the long hours and the huge effect the job had had on my life. I could not believe I had worked so hard, though at the time I just got on with it.

Around the time I was reading my old diaries, junior doctors were being attacked in the news. It was hard for them to tell the public their side of the story, probably because they were too busy working all the time. I thought people should know the truth about what it really means to be a doctor. I wanted to do my bit to stick up for them.

So I decided to share my story. Here are some of the notes I kept during my time in the NHS – the good, the bad and the ugly. They show what it's really like on the wards, the ways the job changed my life, and how one day it all got too much.

Tuesday, 3 August 2004

Day one. My partner, H, has made me a packed lunch. I have a bag full of brand-new doctor's equipment, a new shirt and a new email address. The person who set it up has spelled my name wrong. It is atom.kay@nhs.net. It's good to know that, no matter what happens today, no one can say I'm the most useless person in the hospital. I can blame everything on Atom, whoever he is.

Monday, 30 August 2004

We may not get much free time, but we make up for it in stories about patients. Today over lunch we are telling each other the strange things we have had people complain about. They include itchy teeth and a patient who felt pain in their arm every time they went for a wee. Each story gets a polite laugh.

Then it is Sam's turn. He tells us he saw someone this morning who thought they could only sweat from one half of their face.

He sits back and waits for the laugh, but there's nothing. Until we all say at the same time that it sounds like the sign of a serious lung problem. Sam runs off to make a phone call and get the patient back on the ward. I finish his Twix.

Friday, 10 September 2004

I find it strange that every patient on the ward has a pulse of sixty on their chart, so I go and watch the nurse at work while he's not looking. He feels the patient's pulse, looks at his watch and carefully counts the number of seconds per minute.

Sunday, 17 October 2004

I didn't panic when my patient started spraying blood out of his mouth and onto my shirt. But I didn't know what else to do either. Shove a load of kitchen roll down there?

When my boss arrived, he acted quickly and put a tube down the poor patient's throat. Blood was going everywhere: all over me, my boss, the walls, the ceiling. It was like a nightmare episode of *Changing Rooms*. The sound was the worst part. You could hear the blood choke the man with each breath.

The man did stop bleeding, but for the saddest reason. My boss confirmed the patient's death, wrote in the notes and asked the nurse to tell the family. I changed out of my wet clothes.

So there we go, the first death I've ever seen and every bit as awful as it could have been. My boss took me outside for a cigarette – we both needed one after that. And I don't even smoke.

Tuesday, 9 November 2004

I am called down to the ward at 3 a.m., just as I've closed my eyes for the first time in three shifts. It's to give a sleeping pill to a patient whose need for sleep is apparently more important than mine. I must have magic powers, because I stagger down there only to find the patient has already fallen asleep.

Friday, 12 November 2004

My boss, Henry, has worked out why a patient's blood tests aren't normal. They have been affected by some herbal tablets the patient has been taking to make her feel calmer. Henry explains the side effects and she is shocked. 'I thought they were just made from plants. How dangerous can they be?'

Everyone else in the room goes silent, as Henry sighs. It's clearly not the first time he's heard this from a patient.

'Apricot stones contain poison,' he says. 'The death cap mushroom has a fifty per cent death rate. Plants are not always safe. There is one in my garden where if you simply sat under it for ten minutes you would be dead.' The patient throws away the tablets. Job done.

Later on, I ask him the name of that plant.

'Water lily,' he replies.

Monday, 6 December 2004

I have been asked to fill in a form about the extra hours I've worked this week (not that I will be paid for any of them). I realize I have seen H for less than two hours and worked for a grand total of ninety-seven.

Monday, 31 January 2005

I saved a life tonight. I was called to see an old man who was very close to death. If the vending machine I went to had been working and I'd bought my Mars bar as planned, I might have been too late.

There wasn't time to think about what to do. I just had to act fast. I did what I was trained to do and very soon the man was looking much better. Sorry, Death, better luck next time. By the time Henry arrived, I felt like Superman.

Everyone thinks we go around like superheroes, preventing disasters every day, but it's the first time I've actually saved a life in five months as a doctor. Many lives are obviously saved every day on hospital wards, but almost every time it happens it's down to people working as a team and calmly carrying out a plan.

However, today it was down to me. Henry seems happy, or at least as happy as he ever gets. 'Well,' he says, 'you've bought the man another few weeks on earth.' I bet nobody ever says that to Superman.

Monday, 7 February 2005

Today I saw an injury I will never forget, although I would quite like to. Patient WM is eighteen and was on a night out with friends. At 2 a.m. he was dancing on the roof of a bus shelter and decided to use a lamp post to get back to the ground. He slid down it as though it was a fireman's pole. Unfortunately, the lamp post wasn't smooth at all, so it was a bumpy and extremely painful ride to the pavement. He ended up with deep cuts on both hands . . . and all of the skin and muscle torn off his penis. The medical term is a 'degloving'. It was a bloody mess, to say the least. It made me think of the last piece of pasta stuck to the bowl with a smear of tomato sauce.

WM was upset, and even more so when he asked if the skin could be stuck back on. My boss had to explain that this would be too difficult, since the skin was spread over an eight-foot lamp post in west London.

Monday, 21 February 2005

I sign a patient off work for two weeks, and she offers me £10 to sign her off for a month. I laugh but it's not a joke. She raises her offer to £15.

On the way home, I wonder how much she would have needed to offer before I said yes. £50 would probably do it. I could do with the money, after all.

Monday, 14 March 2005

I go out for pizza with H and some mates. It is one of those places that is trying to be fashionable, with ugly decor and an annoying ordering system. They give you a plastic thing that makes a noise when your order is ready. Then you go and collect your pizza from a bored waiter who will no doubt still expect a tip, even though you've done all the work yourself.

When it goes off I say, 'Oh my God', and jump to my feet. The fucking thing sounds exactly like my hospital alarm.

Monday, 11 April 2005

About to take a ten-year-old to surgery. I watch and learn as Colin, a charming older doctor, deals with the worried mum. He explains what's going on in her son's tummy and how we plan to fix it. He then tells her how long this will take and when the boy will be able to go home.

She seems to relax as he talks. Colin has clearly put her mind at rest. When it is time to take the kid upstairs, Colin nods to the mum and says, 'Quick kiss before he goes?' She leans over and pecks Colin on the cheek. Her son is wheeled away, his own cheek sadly dry.

Thursday, 16 June 2005

I told a patient that he could not have a scan until next week. He was so angry he said he would break both my legs. My first thought was, 'Well, it would be nice to have a couple of weeks off work.' I wondered whether to find him a baseball bat.

Tuesday, 5 July 2005

I'm trying to work out how much alcohol an old lady drinks so I can record it in her notes.

Me: 'And how much wine do you drink per day, would you say?'

Her: 'About three bottles on a good day.'

Me: 'OK . . . And on a bad day?'

Her: 'On a bad day I only manage one.'

Thursday, 7 July 2005

There has been a horrific terror attack in London. All doctors are told to report to A&E.

My job was to send home any patient whose life was not in danger and clear the wards for new arrivals from the bombings. I went round the wards like a steamroller, kicking out anyone who didn't look like they might die. I got rid of hundreds of the fuckers who were using up all of our beds.

Wednesday, 13 July 2005

After the terror attack, the hospital didn't receive any extra patients. Because I was a little, shall we say, keen and sent all my patients home, I have hardly done any work all week.

Saturday, 23 July 2005

This weekend is my best mate Ron's stag do and I have had to cancel at the last minute. I'm sad for him and even sadder for myself. That's £400 I'll never see again, and a T-shirt with Ron's face printed on it that I'll never wear.

I did my best to swap shifts with other doctors, but now one of them has let me down because there is an issue with one of their children. I'm not sure they even have a child. So here I am on the ward, stone-cold sober.

My friends find it hard to see why I have to cancel so often when they make plans in advance. But, sadly, the bastards who make the hospital rota don't care about my social life.

I order a bottle of whisky that I can't afford and send it to Ron to say sorry. We arrange to meet up in two weeks' time, after my run of night shifts, and after the extra hours I had to take on to cover the cost of the stag do.

Friday, 29 July 2005

I spend the night shift feeling like I am on a boat. Water is gushing in and the only thing on hand to bail it out is a mouse's contact lens.

Every patient needs at least fifteen minutes of my time. I am called to see a new one every five minutes so the sums just don't add up. The senior doctors are tied up in a busy A&E, so I deal with the people who sound the sickest first and try to explain to the nurses who call me about other cases.

'I'm really sorry but I've got a load of patients who are much more urgent,' I say. 'It will take me about six hours to get to yours.'

Some of them understand, but some look at me as if I've just said, 'Fuck off, I'm in the middle of watching a box set.' I run from patient to patient all night. Somehow we all get out alive.

At 8 a.m. one of the nurses calls me to say I did really well tonight and she thinks I'm a good little doctor. This makes me sound like a character on CBBC, but it's actually the first time someone has given me any praise since I started the job. Because I am still in shock, I end the call with 'Love you, bye.' My mistake is partly because I'm so tired and partly because H is the only person who ever says nice things to me. But in that moment I really did love the nurse for saying that.

Monday, 8 August 2005

I have had to decide what type of doctor I want to be for the rest of my career. I have chosen to work in women's health, dealing with labour and infertility. What could be a better use of my training than to deliver babies, and help couples who don't seem able to have them? In this area of medicine you tend to end up with twice as many patients as you had at the start, which can only be a good thing. Much better than working with old people, where you eventually end up with none. Of course, working with pregnant women means it is very sad when things go wrong. But the depth of the lows is the price you pay for the height of the highs.

It's my first week working on labour ward. Today I was called in by the midwife because patient DH was feeling unwell soon after the birth of her healthy baby. I had a feeling this might have something to do with the huge amounts of blood DH was losing all over me. I tried to stay calm and tell her everything was going to be fine.

After the worst was over and DH was stable, I went to change into some clean trousers. It's the third time this week that my boxer shorts have been soaked in someone else's blood. Each time I have had to chuck them away and continue the shift with no pants on. My salary barely covers the cost of my underwear!

Saturday, 27 August 2005

A first-year doctor asks me to come and look at a patient who has not had a wee for nine hours. I tell him I haven't had a wee in eleven hours because of people like him wasting my time. His face crumples like a crisp packet in a fat kid's fist, and I feel bad for being mean to him. I was in his position only a few months ago.

The patient is indeed unable to have a wee. It's because the tube (called a catheter) she needs to use is trapped under the wheel of her bed and her bladder is now the size of a space hopper. I stop feeling bad.

Monday, 19 September 2005

I deliver a baby for the first time and suddenly feel like a real doctor. My boss, Lily, talks me through it gently, but I do it all myself. It feels amazing.

'Well done, you did such a great job,' says Lily.

'Thank you!' I reply. Then I realize she was talking to the mum.

Wednesday, 16 November 2005

I glance at the notes before visiting an elderly patient on the ward.

Good news: she has finally been seen by a specialist.

Bad news: the entry reads, 'Patient too sleepy to examine properly.'

I pop in. The patient is dead.

Tuesday, 22 November 2005

I've already helped other doctors with fifteen c-sections. They have offered to let me do the operation myself, but each time I've wimped out. I'm now the only one of the new doctors who's still a virgin, as my boss Ernie is so keen on putting it.

Ernie doesn't give me a choice today. He just tells the patient I am the doctor who is going to deliver her baby. And so I do. I cut through human skin for the first time and deliver a baby through the tummy for the first time. I'd like to say it was amazing, but I had to focus far too hard on every step to take any of it in.

It takes nearly an hour from start to finish, twice as long as it is meant to. Ernie is very kind. He shows me how to write up the notes and takes me out for coffee after. Now I'm no longer a virgin, he tells me, I will get better at it in time. He sounds like some kind of sex pervert. It will get less bloody and less scary and one day will feel routine, he says. Another doctor chips in: 'I wouldn't try to make it last any longer, though.'

Sunday, 25 December 2005

Good news/Bad news.

Good news: it's Christmas morning.

Bad news: I have to work on labour ward.

Worse news: my phone goes off. It's my boss. I didn't set my alarm and they want to know where the hell I am.

Even worse news: I'm asleep in my car. It takes me a while to work out where I am and why.

Good news: it seems I fell asleep after my shift last night and I'm already at work, in the hospital car park. I leap out of the car, grab a quick shower and get there only ten minutes late.

I have eight missed calls from H and a text saying 'Merry Christmas'. No kiss.

This year we are doing Christmas on my next day off: the sixth of January. I tried to be positive about it: 'Just think how cheap the crackers will be by then!'

Friday, 27 January 2006

I have been visiting Baby L on the special care baby unit for three months now. It has become part of my routine before I head home. It's always nice to see a familiar face, even if it is through a glass wall.

He arrived fourteen weeks early and when he was born he weighed less than a jar of jam. His mum was seriously ill and I looked after her for many weeks.

A few decades ago, this baby would have been unlikely to survive, but today his odds are very good. I've watched him change from a tiny scrap of a thing, hooked up to tubes and wires, to a proper screaming, vomiting, and occasionally sleeping, baby.

He's going home this afternoon. I should be pleased, and I am of course, but I'm still going to miss seeing my little pal.

I buy the least hideous card they have in the hospital shop and leave it with the nurses to pass on to the baby's mum. I say how glad I am that their story had a happy ending. I give her my phone number and ask her to text me a picture of the baby every now and again. It is against all the rules, but I'm prepared to break them for this one. And she did text me.

Wednesday, 22 March 2006

It's 3 a.m. Patient RO is twenty-five years old and thirty weeks into her first pregnancy. She complains of a large number of painless spots on her tongue. I inform her they are taste buds.

Monday, 3 April 2006

My night shift is strangely quiet so I go and stare at Facebook for a bit. I comment on how cute a friend's latest ugly baby looks. This comes easily to me, as I spend much of my working day doing the same thing to total strangers. I always find it funny that sensible adults manage to convince themselves that their slimy, squished baby's face is beautiful.

I'm just going through Facebook profiles to make sure everyone I've ever dated is fat and miserable without me, when I see a post pop up. It's from Simon, a school friend's younger brother. His post reads: 'Goodbye everyone. I'm done.'

I realize I might be the only person reading this at 2 a.m. on a Monday. I don't even know Simon that well, but I send him a private message to ask if he is OK. I tell him I'm awake. I remind him that I'm a doctor and I give him my mobile number.

He calls me, drunk and crying. He and his girlfriend have just split up.

I have as much training in this area as I do in laying bathroom tiles. But Simon seems to trust me and that's good enough for both of us.

Two hours later, we've had a good chat. He is going to get a taxi to his mum's house and see his GP in the morning. When we hang up, I get the same rush I feel after any medical emergency. I'm tired but positive and feel like I've done a good thing. I might have made more of a difference to Simon than to any of my patients tonight.

I answer a call from the ward and head down to see a pregnant woman who wants me to look at a mild rash. It's 5 a.m. 'I thought you would be less busy now than in the morning,' she says.

Monday, 19 June 2006

I respond to an urgent call about a woman who has been put into labour because her baby is late. The patient has just been to the toilet and the midwife is extremely worried. The toilet contains an explosion of red and brown liquid. It looks like very bad news for the patient and even worse news for the person who has to clean it up.

I spend the next few hours looking into every possible cause. The baby seems fine and the patient isn't in any pain. In the end, I put in an urgent call to another doctor for advice and the patient goes off for a scan.

Later in the day, the results come back from the specialist doctor. It turns out that the nightmare in the toilet bowl was in fact due to the two large jars of beetroot the patient had eaten the night before. The specialist doctor suggests that next time I want to send him a patient who has the same problem, I taste the contents of the toilet first.

Friday, 21 July 2006

I am called to the ward at 5 a.m. to write up the notes for a patient due to go home in the morning. It should have been done during the day by her own doctor. But if I don't do it, the patient will not be able to go home. I sit down and get on with it, plotting how to get revenge on my colleague.

On my way out, I see that the light is on in a side room, so I pop my head in to check that patient CR is OK. I saw her in A&E last week and have been on night shifts since, so have not heard her news. It turns out she has cancer, and only a few months left to live.

When I saw her in A&E I thought the signs were there but didn't say it. I was taught that if you say the word 'cancer' even once, it is all the patient then remembers. It doesn't matter what else you say or do, to them it feels as though you have said 'cancer cancer cancer' for half an hour.

You never want a patient to have cancer, of course, but I *really* didn't want CR to have it. She was friendly and funny and chatty. It was as if we were two old mates.

She bursts into tears. Her son will graduate from university and she won't be there. Her daughter will get married and she won't be there. She will never meet her grandchildren. Her husband will never get over it. 'He doesn't even know how the boiler works!' She laughs, so I laugh with her. I don't really know what to say. I want to lie and tell her everything is going to be fine, but we both know it won't.

We talk about boring practical things and, as she tells me her worries, I can see it's helping her. It occurs to me that I might be the first person she's been able to open up to about all this. On the way home I phone my mum to tell her I love her.

Wednesday, 2 August 2006

I have started at a new hospital. Junior doctors have to move to a different hospital every six to twelve months. Just as you are getting used to one hospital and making friends with the people who work there, you are moved away to a place full of strangers. It's like the first day of school every time. All junior doctors change hospitals on exactly the same day as each other, which is known as Black Wednesday.

It is a known fact that death rates go up on Black Wednesday. This really takes the pressure off, so I'm not trying very hard.

Wednesday, 16 August 2006

As I delivered a baby today, the midwife on duty with me said I seemed more experienced than I actually am. But her nickname is 'Dangerous Dawn' so I'm not sure she is the best judge.

A phone call from Mum to say my sister Sophie has got into medical school. I send Sophie a text to say well done, then send her a photo of me giving the thumbs-up. 'This will be you in six years!' I write. I crop out the bloodstains on my clothes.

If the call had come at the end of the shift, my text would have said, 'RUN LIKE THE FUCKING WIND.'

Monday, 21 August 2006

I've been carrying a Post Office 'Sorry you were out' card around with me for the last two weeks. I keep taking it out and looking at it like it's a photo of my first child. I would not have time to get to the Post Office and back in my lunch hour, even if I had a lunch hour. Which of course I don't. But I've been hoping I might get off work early one day. Like if the hospital burns down. Or if war breaks out.

The Post Office can only hold on to items for eighteen days, every one of which I've been at work. So the parcel has now been sent back and H won't be getting a birthday present tomorrow.

Wednesday, 27 September 2006

I'm off sick for the first time since I became a doctor. I don't think they will be sending me a Get Well Soon card.

'Oh, for fuck's sake,' said my boss when I called. 'Can't you just come in for the morning?' I explained I had a bad stomach bug and was vomiting so much that I could barely leave the bathroom. 'Fine,' he said. 'But phone around and find someone who's on leave to cover for you.'

I don't know of any other job where you have to arrange your own sickness cover. The North Korean army maybe? How ill would I have to be before someone else had to arrange my cover? A broken leg? A coma?

I always thought that if I ended up off sick, it would be work that caused it. Maybe as a result of getting beaten up by a patient's angry relative, or falling asleep and crashing my car into a tree after yet another night shift. But it was actually because of a lasagne brought in by a patient's mother. I know it can't have been anything else. I was so busy that it was the only thing I had time to eat all day.

Saturday, 7 October 2006

I have now spent six months as Simon's mental health helpline since that first Facebook post. I've told him he can ring me any time he starts to worry, and he does. I've also told him several times to keep seeing his GP, but he doesn't seem to listen to that bit.

Not knowing when the phone is next going to ring with bad news is stressful, and a bit too much like being at work for me. I also know Simon could get better help from someone who didn't have to google 'what to say to someone who wants to kill themselves'. But it seems talking to me is better than nothing. I'm glad he's still here. I panic if I get a missed call from him. What if I call back too late and he's killed himself? Does that make it my fault?

We spoke again this evening. I listened and told him the way he feels will pass. We seem to have the same chat every time, but perhaps it doesn't matter. Simon just wants to know someone cares. I guess that's a big part of what being a doctor is.

Monday, 9 October 2006

Today I heard about a problem so absurd, I looked around the room for hidden cameras. A patient's husband tells me that he can't find any condoms that will fit him. After a long talk I realize this is because he pulls them right down over his balls.

Tuesday, 10 October 2006

I didn't hear what the argument was about but I saw a woman storm out of the room. 'I pay your salary!' she screamed at the nurse. 'Can I have a raise then?' the nurse yelled back.

Tuesday, 31 October 2006

I'm leaving work at 10 p.m. rather than 8 p.m. because a patient had major blood loss after her baby was born. I am meant to be going to a Halloween party but now I don't have time to go home and change into my costume. Would it be so wrong to go straight to the party? After all, I am dressed as a doctor and covered from head to toe in blood . . .

Monday, 29 January 2007

My favourite patient died a couple of weeks ago. I can't stop thinking about her. She was eighty years old and had been on the cancer ward for as long as I've worked here. So I knew it was going to happen at some point.

She was only five feet tall and had bright, smiling eyes. She loved to tell long stories, but she would become bored with telling them just as soon as they got interesting. Almost all of them ended with her saying 'blah, blah, blah' and giving a wave of her hand.

Best of all, she hated my boss. She called him 'old man' every time she saw him, even though he was about fifteen years younger than her. I'd always look forward to seeing her on my shifts. We'd have a good chat and I felt like I'd really got to know her.

Over the months I had met all her children, as well as the many friends who came to visit her. 'NOW they like me!' she would say. Despite the joke, you could see why everyone did.

I was really upset when I heard she had died. I decided to go to the funeral. It felt like the right thing to do. So I swapped my shift with another doctor and let my boss know.

He told me I couldn't go. I know doctors aren't meant to get too close to their patients, but from his tone you would think I was going along to try and sleep with her grandchildren. I guess the real reason doctors aren't meant to go to their patients' funerals is the blame or shame around it. Like the doctor has lost or failed if a patient dies.

Of course, I went to the funeral anyway. I'd already had my suit dry-cleaned, plus I knew how the patient felt about my boss. It was exactly the 'fuck you' she would have wanted. It was a beautiful service and I was glad to be there, for me and for the friends and family I'd met on the ward. Plus, I was able to sleep with one of her grandchildren. (Just kidding!)

Sunday, 4 February 2007

I know everyone moans about how much they get paid and thinks they deserve more. But I really don't think the sums add up for a junior doctor. Your job means making life-and-death decisions every day. You go to medical school for six years. Then you become a doctor, but you have to keep taking exams. You often work over one hundred hours a week. Today I realized that the parking meter outside the hospital is on a better hourly rate than I am.

Monday, 12 February 2007

Today I had to give a patient the morning-after pill. She said, 'I slept with three guys last night. Will one pill be enough?'

Monday, 9 April 2007

I got my exam results today. I have somehow passed the next stage of my medical training and I am in the pub with Ron to celebrate. Sadly, I am only drinking orange juice as I have to head straight off afterwards to do a night shift. They tend to frown on doctors who turn up drunk.

Ron passed his own set of exams last week, so we compare notes. The bank he works for cut down his hours so he could study, but I had to squeeze in as much as my tired eyes would allow after work. Ron had a full month off before the exam. I asked for a week off, but a gap in the rota meant I had to work. Ron had all his exam fees paid for by his company. I had to spend around £300 on books, £500 on a course and £400 on the exam itself. The only upside was I was able to steal the pencil I used to fill in the paper.

Passing his exam means Ron will get a pay rise. All mine means is that I can now enter the next set of exams.

'No,' Ron says wickedly. 'All it means is that you spent over a grand on a pencil.'

Saturday, 5 May 2007

Because I don't get paid enough, I have invented my own bonus. I take home spare uniforms to wear as pyjamas, and sometimes I steal hospital food. It's 1 a.m. I'm very hungry and now is my only chance to get some food for the next seven hours. I head to the kitchen on the ward.

There's a new sign up on the fridge warning staff that meals are for patients only. I ignore it. But then I see the meal tonight is 'Mince with Sultanas'. It's as though they invented the most horrible food they could think of. I'll just take my chances and let nervous energy and Red Bull keep me going.

Tuesday, 12 June 2007

It's five minutes until my shift ends and I need to get away on time to go out for dinner. So, of course, I am asked to see a patient. The midwife looking after her tells me she hasn't been signed off to give the patient the kind of stitches she needs.

Me: 'I haven't been signed off to do them either.'

Midwife: 'You don't need to get signed off to do things – you're a doctor.' (Sad but true.)

Me: 'Isn't there another midwife who can do it?'

Midwife: 'She's on her break.'

Me: 'I'm on my break.' (Not true.)

Midwife: 'You don't get breaks.' (Sad but true.)

Me (begging in a voice I have never heard myself use before): 'But it's my birthday.' (Sad but true.)

Midwife: 'It's labour ward – it's always someone's birthday.'

Tuesday, 26 June 2007

I have been in trouble with H for days now. We were at H's friend Lucy's house. Lucy is pregnant and, just before dinner, she showed us the photos of their recent 3D scans. I think there is no point to 3D scans apart from making the 3D-scan company rich and boring the pants off dinner-party guests. I had a feeling this opinion would go down like a cup of cold sick, so I had a polite look through the pictures along with everyone else.

'Does everything look OK to you?' Lucy asked me. I wanted to say, 'Looks the same as they all fucking do,' but I just smiled. I handed the photos back and said, 'She looks perfect.' There was an icy silence and murder flashed across Lucy's eyes. 'She? SHE?' Oops.

It turned out they had wanted the sex of the baby to be a surprise. This is the first time I've made this mistake. Worst of all, she's a friend, not a patient. Dinner felt like it took a week.

It didn't help that things were already tense at home. Two weeks ago it all went wrong with the flat we were trying to buy. The owners have decided not to sell it after all. I suspect it's more that they don't want to sell it to H and me, but to someone with more money instead.

The whole process has already cost us several thousand pounds in legal fees and surveys. I know more about this flat than I do about any of my closest relatives. But I will never set foot in it again.

By an amazing twist of fate, the couple who own the flat turned up in my clinic today. I had not met them before, but I noticed the address on their notes. The same address that has caused so much stress. If only there was a way I could get my revenge. If this were an action movie, this would be the part where I produce two samurai swords and give a ten-minute speech about honour and respect, before chopping off their heads.

But back in the real world, doctors have to treat you as well as they can, whoever you are. Through gritted teeth I gave them the help they needed. I did the scan and showed them the baby's heart beating. 'It all looks normal,' I said. 'Look, there's an arm. That's a leg. There's his penis . . . Oh, didn't you know? It's a boy.'

Saturday, 30 June 2007

There is a news story in the paper about a hospital porter who has been sent to prison for pretending to be a doctor for the last few years. I have just finished one of those shifts when I wished I could get away with pretending to be a porter.

Monday, 23 July 2007

I tell a patient she can have sex again as soon as she feels ready, but to use protection until her next period. I nod at her husband and say, 'That means HE has to use a condom.' I can't work out why they both look at me in shock. What have I said? It's good advice. I look at them both again and realize the man is her father.

Wednesday, 8 August 2007

Three years into the job, I have now been promoted. When I started out I thought the doctors in this position were always right, like God or Google. I tried never to bother them. As I moved up, I turned to them when I got stuck or needed some wise words. And now the person to turn to is me.

I am often the most senior person in clinic these days. Tradition means I now get called Mr Kay rather than Dr Kay – which makes my ten years of studying so far feel like a fucking waste of time.

I am now in charge of labour ward. There are more senior doctors I can call on in a crisis, but most of the time it's down to me to keep every mum and baby alive. Sometimes there can be a dozen births happening at once. It is as though I am always having to solve a difficult puzzle involving babies and surgical instruments.

It sounds horrific, and at times it is. Working long hours doesn't help. Leaving work at 8 p.m. rather than 10 p.m. means I have put myself before my patients. And when I am home, I'm no fun to be around. Switching off after this kind of work is hard.

But I still go to work with a spring in my step. It feels like everything at work and home is clicking into place. I hope I can keep it that way.

Tuesday, 2 October 2007

I pick up my phone from the locker after a very long day on labour ward. There are seven missed calls from Simon and a bunch of voicemails. I can hardly bear to press play in case it's already too late. It turns out Simon has simply sat on his phone. The little bastard.

Monday, 12 November 2007

All staff have to go to a talk on patient safety. This is because last week a patient had their healthy left kidney taken out, leaving only their useless right kidney. The hospital is very keen that a mistake like this does not happen again. They remind us that in the last three years, British surgeons have drilled holes in the wrong side of patients' skulls fifteen times. Fifteen times a doctor has been unable to tell left from right while holding a drill to your head. Never again will I say something is 'hardly brain surgery'.

The new rule is that any patient going to surgery must have a large arrow drawn in black pen on their left or right leg to show the doctors which side to operate on. I put my hand up and ask what to do if the patient already has a tattoo of an arrow on the wrong leg. Everyone laughs and my boss calls me a fucking clown.

Tuesday, 13 November 2007

I get an email from the hospital management to say that if a patient has a tattoo of an arrow on either leg, it should be covered up with tape and a new arrow drawn in pen on the correct leg. This has now been added to the official rules and they thank me very much for my help.

Saturday, 19 January 2008

I decided to go into work on my Saturday off. 'If you're having an affair you can just tell me, you know,' said H.

I did a big operation yesterday and wanted to make sure the patient was OK. Every time my phone went off this morning, I thought it must be the weekend team telling me something had gone wrong. So I went in to check and to stop myself from going mad.

The patient was fine and had just been seen by another doctor. I didn't want the doctor to think I didn't trust him to do his job properly so I pretended I was 'just passing'. 'I don't blame you for coming in,' the doctor said. He told me he had once been in the same situation after his first ever big operation. He had planned his patient's care to the last detail and been to check on her several times. Then, on the day she was meant to go home, she choked to death on an egg and cress sandwich.

I begin the long drive home and think about what H said earlier. Even if I wanted to have an affair, I think I would be too tired to take off my trousers.

Friday, 29 February 2008

For some reason, a lot of patients insert unusual objects into their bodies during the holidays.

At Christmas I have seen a stuck fairy and a patient who burned her vagina after stuffing a string of lights inside and switching them on. 'I put the Christmas lights up myself' usually has a different meaning.

This is my first leap year working as a doctor and the great British public have not held back.

Patient JB decided to follow tradition and ask her boyfriend to marry her. She bought a ring and put it inside a Kinder Surprise egg. She then put it up her vagina for him to find. The plan was that he would remove it, she would go down on one knee, and then perhaps go down on him too . . .

Sadly, it got stuck and neither of them could get it out. JB was keen to keep it a surprise and would not tell him what she had done or why. But in the end it seemed a good idea to seek help in the hospital. I met them in room three. It was a very easy delivery.

JB had not told me what was inside the egg either. Her boyfriend and I both thought it was very strange when she asked him to open it. I gave him a pair of gloves, which made the whole thing even less romantic.

JB asked her boyfriend to marry her. He said yes, perhaps out of shock or the fear of what she might do if he said no. I wonder where the best man will keep the rings at the wedding?

Thursday, 17 April 2008

Sometimes it's the little things that make a difference on labour ward. The touch on your arm and a quiet thank-you from the new mum too tired to speak. The Diet Coke a nurse buys you because you look so tired. The nod from your boss that says 'you've got this'.

But sometimes it's the really big things that make a difference. A patient's husband takes me to one side after a difficult birth to thank me. He tells me he works for a famous champagne company and wants to take my name so he can send me a gift. I spend a week dreaming about taking a swim in a giant glass of expensive fizz, as if I am a showgirl in Las Vegas.

Today a parcel arrived for me at work. Inside was a baseball cap and key ring. Not quite what I had in mind . . .

Tuesday, 13 May 2008

I go to a pub quiz with Ron and some friends. One of the questions is, 'How many bones are there in the human body?' I get it wrong and the team are very cross with me. I try to explain to them that it's not something you get taught. At no time on the job would you ever need to know this. I wouldn't expect Ron to know how many types of tax there are . . .

It's too late. I can see the look on their faces. They are clearly thinking about all the times they have asked for medical advice from a doctor who doesn't even know how many bones there are in the body. Three other teams get the answer right. (It's 206, by the way.)

Monday, 2 June 2008

Today I was called in by a midwife. Her patient was a healthy woman near the end of her pregnancy. The midwife had been unable to hear the baby's heartbeat. This happens quite often and most of the time everything turns out to be OK.

But I can tell as soon as I walk into the room that something is wrong. The midwife is very pale. The patient and her husband are both doctors and seem to have guessed it won't be good news. Sadly, when we look at the screen we can all see that the baby's heart is no longer beating.

The woman is very calm. She goes into work mode, just like I have to. Her husband is in tears. 'You shouldn't have to bury your child.'

Thursday, 5 June 2008

The rota has been sending me to every corner of the hospital lately. I've given up hope of seeing someone I recognize unless they are handing me a coffee in Costa.

It is very rare to see the same patient more than once, but on labour ward this afternoon I see the doctor from Monday whose baby's heart had stopped. Today, she has to give birth on labour ward.

She and her husband seem strangely pleased to see me. I guess it's because I am a familiar face and I already know what has happened, so they don't have to explain it all again. This must be such a sad and scary time for them.

What the hell can you say? It feels like an awful gap in our training. No one has ever taught us how to speak to couples who have lost a child. Will I make it better or worse if I say something hopeful about 'next time'? Do I say how sad I feel for them? How about a hug?

Stick to what you know. I just talk to them about what is going to happen next. They have a lot of questions which I do my best to answer.

I pop back every hour or so to see how they are doing. It goes past 8 p.m. and I decide to stay until it has happened.

H is waiting for me at home, but I lie in a text and say there has been an emergency and I need to stay. I don't know why I can't just tell the truth. I lie to the patient too when she asks why I am still here after 11 p.m. 'I have to cover for someone,' I say. It does feel like my being here is helping them a bit.

The baby is born soon after midnight. I talk through the tests we can do to find the cause of death. They want me to do them all, which means I have to take skin and blood samples from the baby. This is the worst thing I have to do in this job. I used to get so upset that I couldn't look as I did it. Now I can look, but I still find it extremely sad. We expect babies to look beautiful and perfect, but often they don't. I think he must have been dead for a couple of weeks. 'I'm sorry,' I say to him as I take the samples I need. 'There we go. All done now.'

I dress him. Then I look up to a God I don't believe in and say, 'Look after him.'

Tuesday, 10 June 2008

The police stop me on my drive home. 'Did you know you just went through a red light there, sir?' I had no idea. It was a very tough night shift and I'd had no sleep. I hope I was paying more attention to my patients than I was to the road.

I explain that I have been working on a labour ward for the past thirteen hours. They don't seem to give a shit. They give me a £60 fine and three points on my licence. Bastards.

Monday, 7 July 2008

An urgent call to a room on labour ward. The husband was messing around on a birthing ball and fell off, cracking his head on the floor.

Tuesday, 8 July 2008

There are always highs and lows in this job, but I've never seen things take such a sudden turn. I am called to the Early Pregnancy Unit to confirm the loss of a baby at eight weeks. The doctor on duty has not done many scans before and wants a second pair of eyes. I remember that feeling very well, so I rush over. He has clearly made the couple aware that it does not look good. They are sad and silent as I walk in.

It turns out that the doctor may as well have been doing a scan of the back of his hand or a packet of crisps. Not only is the baby fine, but so is the twin he didn't spot. I'm not sure I've ever had to break good news before.

Thursday, 10 July 2008

Next week H and I will head off for a two-week holiday to celebrate five years together. I can't wait to be on a beach on the other side of the world from labour ward. I just hope I haven't forgotten how to be in a relationship that isn't kept alive by text messages that say 'sorry'.

Today, I get an email that tells me I have to work the middle weekend of our holiday. No one else can swap with me, and I don't know how to deliver a baby over Skype.

I know other doctors who have had to come home early from their honeymoon, or miss a family funeral, so I know they won't change the rota for my holiday. Their best suggestion is I just pop 6,000 miles back to England for the weekend.

Thursday, 11 September 2008

I almost cry at the end of a tough night shift when I open a lovely card from a patient. I remember her well.

I gave her some stitches down below after she had her baby a few weeks ago.

> Dear Adam,
> I just wanted to say thank you. You did a great job. My GP checked my stitches and said you could hardly tell I'd had a baby! Thank you so much again.

I am very touched. It's the kind of thing that makes the whole job feel worth it. She has even made the card herself. It's a beautiful white card with her baby's footprint in gold paint on the front. Though perhaps she didn't have much choice. There can't be many cards in Sainsbury's that say, 'Thanks for mending my arsehole!'

Tuesday, 16 September 2008

A woman is very cross that three or four people who arrived on the ward after her have been seen before her. 'If I ever have to go to hospital, madam,' one of the midwives calmly tells her, 'I want to be seen last. Because that means everyone else is sicker than me.'

Thursday, 18 September 2008

My phone rings at 8 p.m. I try to guess if it's because I forgot to turn up for a night shift or because someone else did and they need me to cover. I'm happy to hear it is just my friend Lee, though he does sound rather worried. This is unusual for Lee. He is usually very calm. He works as a lawyer, and I have heard him on the phone talking to the police, saying things like 'Was the whole body destroyed by the acid or just the skull?'

He asks if I am free to come over. His flatmate, Terry, has hurt himself and Lee thinks he should go to hospital, but he would like my advice. It's not far away so I pop round.

Terry has indeed hurt himself. He cut his thumb opening a can of beans. There is blood all over the floor and the top of his thumb is flapping open like a Muppet's mouth. I can even see the bone.

My advice is to get to hospital as fast as possible. I don't think many people in the world would disagree with me on this point. But, sadly, Terry is one of them.

Lee takes me into the kitchen for a chat. Terry really does not want to go to hospital. He drinks a lot and is worried that any blood tests will show problems with his liver.

I spend some time trying to talk Terry into going to hospital. I tell him the doctors will only focus on the fact that half his thumb is hanging off. But Terry still says no. He won't even let me call an ambulance so they can come to the flat and take a look.

Lee and I come up with a new plan while Terry ruins some more tea towels. Lee has a first-aid kit left over from a trip to Africa. He opens it and asks if I have what I need to sew Terry back up. He clearly spent a lot of money on that kit. It contains all the equipment I would need to take out a lung.

After a short time going through the kit, like an auntie trying to find the coffee cream in a box of Milk Tray, I find what I need. The only thing missing is something to take the pain away. Lee jokes that Terry can just bite down on a wooden spoon.

Five minutes later I find myself fixing Terry's wound at the kitchen table. Terry is oddly happy about it. I clean the cut and put in some big stitches to try to stop the bleeding. When the pain gets too much for Terry, he starts to scream. We really don't want to have to explain it all to the people next door. Lee hands Terry the wooden spoon.

I am quite pleased with how the thumb looks when the job is done. I don't know if Terry will listen to my advice on keeping it clean and taking out the stitches. But I tell him anyway. Terry thanks me and gets himself a drink. He says he will never eat beans again.

Thursday, 16 October 2008

It's time to go home. The doctor on the night shift has come from a different hospital to fill a gap in the rota. We have not had a break all day, and it won't be a quiet night either. I tell the new doctor how sorry I am. Busy shifts are even more difficult when you aren't used to the hospital. I can see panic behind his eyes, but he says nothing.

I explain a few things and tell him it will be fine, but he still looks scared. He asks if he will have to do any c-sections. He says he has never done one before.

I wait for him to tell me this is a joke. Maybe he has turned up on the wrong ward and the doctor who actually knows how to work on a labour ward is about to walk in. But no. This guy said yes to taking this job, but no one bothered to ask him if he had worked on a labour ward before.

I send him home and call my boss to ask what to do. I can already guess that the answer will mean me working another twelve hours for free.

Tuesday, 18 November 2008

Ron called to ask me for some advice this evening. His dad has lost a lot of weight and is in terrible pain. He gives me some other details and asks what I think is going on.

If I was being asked on an exam paper, I would say it was a form of cancer with little chance of a cure. If I was being asked by a patient, I would say it was very serious and we needed to do more tests quickly.

But it's different when I am asked by someone close to me. I said it sounded like his GP was doing all the right things (true). I said it still could be nothing (sadly, not true). I knew it was going to be bad news, but really wanted everything to be OK. Ron is my best friend and I have known his dad since I was eleven. You never lie to your patients to give them false hope. But there I was, telling my mate that it would all be fine.

Doctors are always told not to give medical advice to friends and family. But I have always ignored that and given them a private helpline. My job makes me such a useless friend in many ways, so I feel like I have to offer something so as to stay on their Christmas card list. And this is exactly why they tell us not to.

Thursday, 20 November 2008

In no other job would you be expected to share shoes on a 'first come, first served' basis. It is like being at a Megabowl where people get blood everywhere and no one cleans up afterwards.

If you want your own white leather hospital shoes, they cost around £80. So it used to be only the bosses who had them. They would glide around the hospital like they had two giant paracetamols on their feet.

But now there is a new kind of shoe called Crocs. They come in bright colours, they do the same job and they cost less than £20. They also have holes in them, so you can lock your shoes together with a padlock and no one else will get their hands on them.

Today there is a sign in the changing rooms. It says: 'Staff must not wear Crocs shoes as the holes will not protect feet from falling needles.' Someone has added a note in pen: 'And they make you look like a dick.'

Saturday, 10 January 2009

It was Pete and Mary's wedding today. None of us could believe that two doctors would both be able to get their big day off work. One of my friends only got the afternoon of her wedding day off. She had to do the morning clinic in full hair and make-up so as to make it to the church on time.

The really amazing thing is that they have managed to stay together at all. The hospital system isn't great for anyone's love life. Pete and Mary got their first jobs in different parts of the country. This meant they spent the next five years working 120 miles apart. Pete had to move to a different house to be near his job and pop back home when the rota let him. Which it mostly didn't.

The best man at the wedding was also a doctor. He gave a brilliant speech, saying Pete and Mary's relationship was like dating an astronaut who works on the International Space Station. He had to do the speech between the starter and the main course and then dash off for a night shift.

Thursday, 29 January 2009

I had to wait for about a minute during a c-section until Heart FM had moved on to the next song. Cutting Crew might be the perfect band name for during an operation, but I refuse to deliver a baby to the chorus of 'I just died in your arms tonight'.

Saturday, 7 February 2009

I missed the first half of a musical called *Les Mis* thanks to a difficult birth which kept me at work late. I had no idea what was going on in the second half. It didn't help that the good guy and the bad guy had very similar names.

I went to the pub with Ron and the others after the show. Watching the first half didn't seem to have helped anyone else understand it either.

Sunday, 8 February 2009

Simon rang me to say he had cut his wrists last night after a fight with his new girlfriend. He ended up in hospital, though he was back at home now and feeling OK.

He asked if I was angry with him, and I said of course not. I was actually very angry that he hadn't called me first so I could try and calm him down. Surely he owed me that much? I felt bad that I hadn't done enough or been able to stop him doing it. And then I felt bad about being so angry with him.

We talked for an hour or so. I told him again that he could call me any time, day or night. We've had the same chat many times in the last few years. I'm sad that things seem no better now than when he put that first cry for help on Facebook.

But maybe that's the wrong way to look at it. It's not like fixing a broken leg. Simon's feelings aren't easy to cure, but he is learning how best to manage them. I should be pleased he's gone this long without something worse happening.

Tuesday, 17 February 2009

The emergency buzzer goes off and causes panic. As well as the usual number of people rushing in, there is dust and rubble everywhere. If this was an episode of *Casualty*, there would be half an ambulance smashed into the room with us, but no. It turns out the midwife pulled the cord so hard she has taken down most of the ceiling.

Wednesday, 4 March 2009

It should not be a rare event for me to leave work on time, but today I manage it. I am going out for dinner with my grandma. After we have eaten our starters she leans over, licks her finger and wipes a bit of food off my cheek. Then she licks her finger again. I realize too late that it was actually a patient's blood. I decide not to say anything.

Saturday, 7 March 2009

'Doctor Adam! You delivered my baby!' cries the woman behind the cheese counter in the supermarket. I have no memory of her at all but I guess she must be right. She knows my name, after all. I ask about 'the little one', because I can't remember if she had a boy or a girl. It was a boy and he's doing well. She asks me all sorts of questions about things we must have talked about while she was in labour. I feel bad that she can remember so much more about me than I can about her. But I guess that while it was one of the biggest days of her life, I might have delivered six other babies on that shift.

'I'll put it through as Cheddar,' the woman whispers to me as she weighs my goat's cheese. It will save me a couple of quid. You don't often get a bonus in this job so it's quite exciting. I smile at her.

'That's not Cheddar,' says her boss, as he walks past. There goes my bonus.

Friday, 3 April 2009

I'm having a drink with Ron. He has decided it's time to move on to a better job. Sometimes I think about moving on myself, but it's hard to know how. There are plenty of different banks for Ron to work in, but only one NHS.

Ron says I must have many skills that could be put to good use in a different job. People who have never worked as doctors always say this. Our training is very specific. I know how to solve some problems, but not all of them. I'm not sure I would be very good at managing a branch of Ryman, for example. What other job could I find that would involve pulling babies and Kinder Eggs out of people?

Monday, 4 May 2009

Another busy day on labour ward. I go to help out with a difficult birth, but when I get there things seem to be going well. I hand over to the midwife and wait at the back of the room just in case they need me. We can soon see the top of the baby's head.

The dad is down there watching. He is very excited and tells his wife how well she is doing. The midwife tells the mum to stop pushing so she can help the baby out slowly. If she stays calm, she won't need stitches.

As the baby's head appears, the dad screams, 'Oh my God! Where is its face?' Mum also screams and the baby's head shoots out. I explain to them that babies are normally born face down.

The baby's face looks perfect, even though there is now blood all over it. I put on some gloves and prepare to sew the mum back up.

Thursday, 25 June 2009

I am down in A&E around 11 p.m. and looking at Twitter while waiting for the next patient. A big news story is breaking. 'Oh my God,' I say. 'Michael Jackson's dead!' One of the nurses sighs and stands up. 'Which room is he in?'

Tuesday, 28 July 2009

I am booking a couple in for a c-section and they ask if they are able to choose the date. They are British Chinese, and I know that in the Chinese calendar some days are lucky and some are unlucky. I say we will do our best to give them a choice. They ask me to check for the first or second of September.

'Are these lucky dates?' I ask. I should get some kind of medal for being so understanding and sensitive.

'No,' the husband says. 'September babies go into a different school year and do better in their exams.'

Monday, 10 August 2009

Yes, madam, you will shit during labour. Yes, it is normal. No, there is nothing I can do to stop it. Although if you had asked me yesterday, I would have said that the massive curry you ate to 'bring on labour' was probably not a good idea.

Wednesday, 18 November 2009

I go to visit Ron's dad in hospital. He looks terrible. He has lost even more weight and is all skin and bone. I can see how hard his body is fighting the cancer, but it has no chance.

'I wish people didn't have to see me like this,' he says. 'It's going to cost a fortune for them to make me look nice for the funeral.'

The doctors are doing all they can to make him comfortable. Ron's dad used to work as an engineer and is amazed by all the machines around him. 'This would not have been possible twenty years ago,' he says, and we talk about how lucky we are to live in the modern world.

'Do you think they will be able to cure cancer twenty years from now?' he asks. I can't work out whether it would be best to say yes or no. 'I only know about vaginas, I'm afraid,' I say, and he laughs.

Then he says, 'Why do we always say that people have lost their battle with cancer? We never say that cancer won the battle against them.' He keeps making jokes, just like he always has. I had been nervous about seeing Ron's dad, but I find I am really enjoying it.

It is kind of him to act like this. It makes things easier for his friends and family, of course. But it also means everyone will remember him as he always was.

Thursday, 10 December 2009

Today I delivered a baby for a mum I saw in the clinic a while ago, when I first started working at this hospital. At the time she was worried she might not ever be able to have children and now here we are. I feel like holding the baby up above my head and singing 'Circle of Life'.

While I sew her up I ask how the treatment I had arranged for her had gone. It turns out she got pregnant without any help the week after she was in my clinic. I'm still calling it a win.

Thursday, 17 December 2009

Sadly, mothers and babies die every year in this country as a result of violence at home. Every doctor has a duty to look out for it. This can be difficult as controlling husbands often go to the clinic with their wives, which stops them from speaking out.

Our hospital has a plan to help women get help if they need it. In the ladies' toilet there is a sign that says: 'If you want to talk about violence at home, put a red sticker on the front of your notes.' There are sheets of red stickers in every toilet.

Today, a woman has put a few red stickers on the front of her notes. It is the first time I have had to deal with this. I find it difficult as her husband and two-year-old child have both come with her. I try but fail to get the husband to leave the room. In the end I call in a midwife to help me and eventually we are able to speak to the woman on her own.

We talk to her gently, but it doesn't seem to help. She seems scared and confused. After ten minutes we realize what has happened. The red stickers were put on the notes by her two-year-old when they went to the toilet together.

Friday, 8 January 2010

More than once I have thought about leaving this job. Some days things go wrong, patients complain or the rota changes at the last minute and it all makes me feel like I've had enough. But I always think how lucky I am to play such a big part in people's lives.

Today, I went to my old school to give some career advice to the pupils. I had to sit behind a table, and dozens of other employers sat behind their own tables.

They all had lots of leaflets and sweets. One company was even giving out doughnuts. I had nothing. When the gangly teenagers asked what it's like to be a doctor, I felt I had to tell them the truth. The hours are terrible, the pay is terrible, you don't get much praise and sometimes you actually feel unsafe. But there is no better job in the world.

It's hard to explain how special it feels to help a couple get pregnant after years of trying and nearly giving up hope. Labour ward is madly busy: rushing from room to room helping any baby who gets sick or gets stuck. But the parents will never forget you.

I can see the appeal of other careers that pay shit-loads of cash, but there is no feeling like knowing you have just saved a life. You go home late and tired and covered in blood, but feel like you have played a useful part in the world.

I said this speech about thirty times. It was like therapy for me. I felt happy as I left the school hall, partly because I took a free doughnut. I'm even looking forward to getting back onto labour ward.

Sunday, 14 February 2010

It is the first Valentine's Day I have spent with H in four years. I joke that going out with a doctor is a bit like having a birthday on the 29th of February.

We have a lovely dinner at a Thai restaurant. At the

end of the meal, the waiter brings over a beautiful wooden box with two sweets in the shape of hearts. I eat mine whole. It turns out it was actually a candle.

Tuesday, 16 February 2010

A husband and wife are in tears when I tell them that the woman will need a c-section. The husband is very keen to be the first person to touch the baby and he won't stop going on about it. There is not much time to wonder why. Does he need to break a magic spell or give the baby some kind of special powers?

He asks if he can be the one to lift the baby out. I know for a fact that he would either faint, vomit or both if he saw inside his wife. It is never a pretty sight.

It also takes most doctors quite a lot of practice before they can take a baby out by the head. Unless the husband wants to go and try scooping melons out of a swamp with one hand for practice, it might be best if he leaves the job to us. We don't even have time to get him dressed up in a gown and gloves. Gloves! That gives me an idea.

'How about if we pass the baby straight to you?' I say. 'We will all be wearing gloves so you will still be the first person to touch her.' He agrees. Problem solved!

Saturday, 27 March 2010

I spend the evening with a few old friends from medical school. It is nice to catch up, even though we had to set a new date about seven times before we could all make it.

After dinner we end up in the medical school bar, for old times' sake. For some reason we start playing drinking games. The only game we can remember is 'I have never'. It turns into a kind of therapy. All six of us have cried because of work. Five of us have cried while at work. All of us have felt unsafe during a shift. Three of us have had relationships end because of work. All of us have missed important family events.

On the plus side, three of us have had sex with nurses and one of us has done this at work. So it's not all bad.

Monday, 19 April 2010

One of the senior doctors, Dr Brown, has taken two weeks off because her dog has died. People are laughing about it in the labour ward coffee room. To my surprise, I find myself telling them not to give her a hard time.

Dr Brown hated me from the moment we met. Once I asked her if I could leave work on time for a birthday dinner with H. Dr Brown said no, and told me I would find it easier to get a new partner than a new job. A few years ago she told me I could not speak to patients about their diet unless I lost some weight myself. She has told me off for all kinds of small things and shouted at me in front of patients.

And yet I am still telling people not to be unkind about her. Why make fun of someone for being upset? We should feel sorry for her. Her pet clearly meant a lot to her and death is sad for everyone.

The others say they suppose I'm right and I walk off feeling like a saint. Two weeks off for a dead dog, though. She must be fucking mad.

Saturday, 5 June 2010

I am so tired these days that I often wake up and have no idea where I am. Today I hear a loud knock and open my eyes. An old man is tapping on the window with his umbrella and asking if I am OK. I seem to have fallen asleep in my car while waiting at a red light.

I almost fell asleep earlier while sitting on a stool, waiting for a patient. We are always told not to use empty hospital rooms to get some sleep during night shifts. But that big ball of fire in the sky always makes it rather hard to sleep during the day. And it is not easy to keep switching from sleeping at night and working in the day to the other way round again.

We are told that we are here to work and not sleep, so we have to stay awake for all of our shift. But surely doctors can do a better job if they have a quick nap when things are quiet? If the boss or his wife needed an emergency operation at 7 a.m., I bet they would not want it done by someone who had been forced to stay awake all night.

It's strange being this tired. You're not all there. I worry that I can't react fast enough. It's like I have had three pints in the pub. And yet if I turned up at work drunk, they would probably send me home.

I left work at 9.30 this morning. It took me an hour to write up my notes because I could not find the words. It was like trying to write them in French. I wonder if the police will take my tiredness as an excuse when, one of these days, I fall asleep at the wheel and run someone over as I drive home.

Friday, 11 June 2010

I tell a pregnant woman that she has to give up smoking. She looks at me like I've just said, 'I want to kill your cat.' She refuses to go to a class that would help her to quit. I explain how bad smoking is for her baby, but she doesn't seem to care. She tells me all her friends smoked when they were pregnant and their kids are fine.

I'm tired and just want to go home. I look at the clock. It is half past six. Clinic was meant to end an hour ago, and she is far from the last patient on my list. I snap.

'If you don't stop smoking when you're pregnant, then nothing will ever stop you and you will die of lung disease!' I know I should not have said this and tell her I'm sorry. But, strangely, it seems to help. She asks me to tell her more about the classes. It's good to know that death threats can work on patients sometimes.

On her way out she jokes, 'Maybe I'll start taking drugs instead!' I laugh and decide not to say that this would probably be safer for the baby than smoking.

Tuesday, 27 July 2010

Ron tried to dump me as a friend today. He doesn't know why he bothers trying to keep in touch with me. It's clear our lives have taken different paths since we were at school together.

He says I use my job as an excuse all the time. I missed his stag do and the first half of his wedding because of work. I missed his dad's funeral because of work. And then his daughter's christening. He knows my job is busy, but how hard can it be to swap a shift for something you really want to do?

I put my hand on my heart and swear to Ron that I love him. He's one of my best friends and I would never lie to him. I know I've been a rubbish friend, but I have still seen a lot more of him than almost anyone else I know. The job is just very busy: it doesn't stop.

No one else can ever really understand how hard it is to be a doctor, or how much it affects your life. I did lie about the christening, though. Fuck that.

Monday, 2 August 2010

It's my last shift in this hospital. A night shift, of course. My new job starts an hour before this one is due to end, and is about ten miles away. I guess I am going to be late.

I am on the stairs at 12.10 a.m. when my swipe card refuses to let me back onto the ward. This job was meant to end at midnight, and I realize the card must have been cut off as soon as the clock struck 12. I am basically Cinderella in scrubs.

If you ask a hospital to provide enough staff, or chairs, or a fast computer, then they will be useless. But when it comes to locking you in and out of wards, they suddenly find a way. I spend the next fifteen minutes banging on the doors and praying no one dies before someone spots me and lets me back on the ward.

Monday, 9 August 2010

A patient named their baby after me today. After I delivered it, I said, 'Adam's a good name,' and the parents agreed.

I say 'Adam's a good name' after every single birth and this was the first time that anyone has ever said yes. I've not even had a middle name before. Once I have enough Adams named after me, maybe I can ask them to work my shifts instead of me.

The student helping me asked how many babies I have delivered. I guessed around 1,200. He then looked up some facts and told me that nine babies out of every 1,200 born in the UK are called Adam. So it would seem that out of nine sets of parents intending to name their child Adam, I have managed to put off eight of them.

Wednesday, 25 August 2010

An eighty-five-year-old cancer patient broke my heart yesterday. She told me she misses her dead husband. Her children have not been to visit since she has been in hospital. And she can't even have her usual bedtime drink of whisky in here.

I decided to do a good deed. I added whisky to her drug chart and gave one of the nurses £20 to get a bottle from the supermarket.

This morning the nurse told me the patient would not take the drink because 'Jack Daniel's tastes like fucking cat piss.'

Friday, 24 September 2010

The emergency alarm sounds. It's Friday night and five minutes before I am due to go home.

Tonight is date night. I am meant to be taking H somewhere very expensive to make up for the fact that I have had to work for the last six date nights. I should be fine if I leave by 6 p.m., I tell myself. It is 5.45 and my patient needs an operation.

There are two ways of dealing with this. The first way – keyhole surgery – will take over an hour of my time, but the patient will be more comfortable and can go home tomorrow. The second way – a normal operation – will take a matter of minutes, but the patient will end up with a scar and will need to stay in hospital for a few days. The second way will mean I get to go home on time and keep H happy. And maybe the patient likes hospital food?

I pause for a moment and then decide to do the right thing. Good news for the patient, bad news for me.

Monday, 11 October 2010

I get a text from Simon. I've not heard from him for the last eighteen months so I worry when I see his name pop up. He is asking for my address as he wants to invite me to his wedding. I'm touched that he thought of me. I look forward to saying yes, and then having to cancel at the last minute due to work.

Thursday, 14 October 2010

The first time a patient started texting while I was doing a smear test, I found it quite weird. But now it happens all the time. Today a patient did a FaceTime call with her friend while I was down there.

Monday, 8 November 2010

I have just had the night shift from hell. We were short of staff and I ran from one crisis to another all night. I lost count of the number of babies I delivered in the end.

I don't think I have ever been this tired. I have not shut my eyes or sat down for twelve hours. My dinner is still in my locker, and I just called a midwife 'Mum' by mistake.

I do one last emergency c-section. The baby is limp, but gets some urgent care and is soon making the right noises. I sew up the patient, feeling glad it has all ended well.

After I leave the room, another doctor grabs me and says I have cut the baby's cheek. I must have done it with the knife when I cut open the mum. It's not a bad cut but they had to let me know.

I go straight back in to see the baby and its parents. The cut won't leave a scar but it was still my fault. I tell the parents how sorry I am. They are in love with their beautiful little girl and say they understand. They know she had to come out in a hurry and these things happen.

I want to say that these things aren't meant to happen. I've not done anything like this before and I don't think it would have happened at the start of the shift, when I was less tired.

I give the parents a leaflet that tells them how to write and complain. But they don't want it. It's a relief for me, but I keep thinking about the poor baby. A little higher and I could have taken her eye out. A little deeper and I could have caused a scar and major blood loss. Babies have even died this way in the past.

I write up the notes and fill in a form. Soon I will be sat down and told off about this. But no one will stop and think about the real problem. These long hours are dangerous for staff and patients alike.

Thursday, 18 November 2010

I was meant to be home at 7 p.m., but it is now 9.30 p.m. and I have only just left labour ward. It seems fitting that work means I have to text H and cancel picking up all my stuff from the house. We have now broken up and I'm living in a tiny little flat. One good thing: at least it's only ten minutes away from the hospital.

Monday, 22 November 2010

A patient in A&E with mild stomach pain has sunk lower and lower down my to-do list this afternoon. Labour ward is very busy today. I am in the middle of seeing a patient who is seriously ill when I get a call from an angry doctor in A&E.

'If you don't come here right now, this patient is going to break our four-hour target,' he says.

'OK,' I say. 'But if I do come right now, my current patient is going to die.'

He is silent for a good five seconds. Which is time neither of us can really afford to waste.

'Fine. Just come when you can,' he snaps. 'But I am really not happy about this.' When my seriously ill patient feels better, I must ask her to write an apology.

Sunday, 5 December 2010

It is Sunday afternoon on labour ward. I am working with an excellent junior doctor. She asks me to look at a patient and I agree that she will need a c-section. The baby is clearly in distress. They are a lovely couple and only got married last year. It's their first baby. They understand when we tell them what needs to be done.

The junior doctor asks if she can do the c-section while I help her. She begins to cut through the skin and then the layers beneath. When she cuts into the womb, there is a huge amount of blood.

I stay calm and ask the junior doctor to deliver the baby. She says she can't because there is something in the way. I take over. I soon realize there is something seriously wrong. It should have been picked up when the patient had her pregnancy scans. She should never have been allowed to go into labour.

I deliver the baby. But the baby is dead. The baby doctors try to save it but, sadly, they can't.

The patient is losing a lot of blood. One litre. Two litres. Nothing I try will stop it. I call for urgent help. We are doing all we can and the husband has been sent out of the room.

She has now lost five litres of blood. I am holding her womb tightly in both hands to try to stop the bleeding.

My boss arrives and tries to help but nothing works. I see panic in her eyes. We are told there is now a chance that the patient's organs will be damaged. We wait for the most senior doctor to arrive. He has no choice but to remove the patient's womb. The patient has now lost twelve litres of blood.

The patient is moved to Intensive Care and I am told to expect the worst. My boss talks to the husband. I start to write up my notes, but instead I just cry for an hour.

After

That was the last diary entry I wrote, and the reason there aren't any more jokes in this book.

Everyone at the hospital was very nice to me. They said all the right things. They told me it wasn't my fault and that I could not have done anything more. I got sent home for the rest of the shift.

A number of people asked if I was OK. But everyone still expected me to come into work the next day and carry on as though nothing had happened. No one was unkind about it. It's just a problem that comes with the job. You can't wear black every time something goes wrong. You can't take a month off to recover. Bad things happen too often. And there is not even enough space in the rota for anyone to take a sick day.

It is difficult for doctors to admit just how badly terrible things like this affect them. The only way to survive is to tell yourself that it is all just part of the job.

I had seen babies die before. I had seen patients die before. But this was different. It was the first time I was the most senior person on the ward when something awful happened. I was the person everyone turned to, and I failed.

I had not broken any of the rules or done anything wrong. Other doctors would have done exactly the same things with exactly the same result. But this wasn't good enough for me. I kept wondering what might have happened differently. I might have prevented this tragedy. It was hard to think about anything else.

I went back to work the next day. I was in the same skin, but I was a different doctor. I knew I could not risk anything bad ever happening again. If a baby's heart rate dropped even a tiny bit, I would do a c-section. I knew this meant women were having c-sections they didn't really need. But if everyone got out of the room alive, it was worth it.

In the past I had not understood why my bosses were afraid of taking risks. But now I could see why. They had all been through something that left them thinking about what might have been. And this was how you dealt with it.

Except I wasn't really dealing with it. I was just getting on with it. In the next six months I didn't laugh once. My smiles weren't real. I was broken by this experience.

I should have been able to talk to someone. In fact, the hospital should have made sure of it. But there is a code of silence that keeps help from those who need it most.

No matter how hard I tried, I knew another terrible thing would happen at some point in the future. There is no way to avoid it. One senior doctor tells her students that by the time they retire there will be a bus full of dead kids and kids with brain damage, and that bus is going to have their name on the side. She tells them that if they can't deal with this then they are in the wrong job.

Maybe if someone had said that to me a bit earlier, I would have thought twice about becoming a doctor. Maybe I would not have become a doctor at all.

I asked if I could go part-time but they said no, not unless I was pregnant. I thought about becoming a GP instead. But it would mean I would have to start my training from scratch, and I didn't know if I even wanted to be a GP.

A few months later, I hung up my white coat. I was done.

I didn't tell anyone why I left. Maybe I should have. They might have understood. When I told my parents, they looked at me as though I'd just said I was going to prison.

At first, it was something I couldn't talk about. But then it became something I just didn't talk about. I would simply change the subject and tell some funny stories about things patients had said or done. Some of my closest friends will read this book and hear that sad story for the first time.

These days I work as a writer. A bad day at work now is when my laptop crashes or I get a bad review – things that really don't matter at all. I don't miss the doctor's version of a bad day. But I do miss the good days. I miss the other doctors I worked with and I miss helping people. I miss that feeling on the drive home that you have made a difference to someone's life.

I have learnt that you never really stop being a doctor. You still run to help if you see someone come off their bike. You still reply to texts from pregnant friends who need advice.

In 2016, the government started forcing doctors to work harder than ever for less money than ever. I knew I had to stand up for the doctors. There were MPs who lied again and again, and said that doctors were being greedy. This made me angry because I knew it wasn't true. Doctors only ever care about the best interests of their patients.

Unfortunately, the junior doctors lost their battle. The government's loud voice drowned out their very quiet one. I suddenly realized that everyone who works for the NHS needs to shout about what their work is really like. Next time a government minister lies and says doctors are just in it for the money, we need the public to know that this is nonsense.

Why would anyone do that job for anything other than good reasons? I wouldn't wish the job on anyone. I have a lot of respect for those who work on the front line of the NHS, because in the end it was too much for me.

I wrote this book six years after I quit. When I meet up with doctors I used to work with, their stories from hospitals still show the NHS in a sad state. When I left, it was very rare for a doctor to change career. Now it happens extremely often. The job is so stressful and so difficult these days that they often move abroad or work in the City. These same doctors were the ones who used to do anything for the job. They would even miss the morning of their own wedding day.

The other thing I notice when I speak to doctors now is how everyone remembers the sad stuff and the bad stuff so clearly. They can remember every detail and their voices shake when they talk about it.

I'm not here to tell their stories, though. That's not what this book is about. It is simply one doctor's point of view. I hope it will give a glimpse of what the job really involves.

But promise me this. The next time an MP attacks the NHS, don't just accept what they try to feed you. Think about the toll the job takes on every doctor, nurse and midwife. Think about what they must go through at home and at work. Don't forget that they do an impossible job and try to do their very best every day. Your time in hospital may well hurt them a lot more than it hurts you.

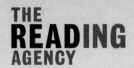

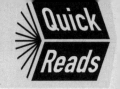

About Quick Reads

"Reading is such an important building block for success"

- Jojo Moyes

Quick Reads are short books written by best-selling authors. They are perfect for regular readers and adults reading for pleasure for the first time. Since 2006, over 4.8 million copies of more than 100 titles have been read!

Available to buy in paperback or ebook and to borrow from your local library.

Turn over to find your next Quick Read...

A special thank you to Jojo Moyes for her generous donation and support of Quick Reads and to **Here Design**.

Quick Reads is part of The Reading Agency, a national charity tackling life's big challenges through the proven power of reading.

www.readingagency.org.uk

@readingagency   #QuickReads

The Reading Agency Ltd. Registered number: 3904882 (England & Wales)
Registered charity number: 1085443 (England & Wales)
Registered Office: Free Word Centre, 60 Farringdon Road, London, EC1R 3GA
The Reading Agency is supported using public funding by Arts Council England.

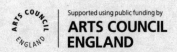

Supported using public funding by

**ARTS COUNCIL
ENGLAND**

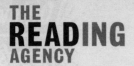

Find your next Quick Read:
the 2020 series

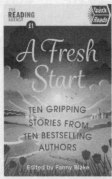

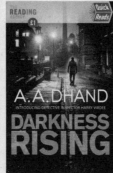

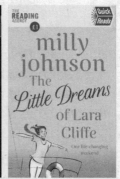

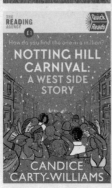

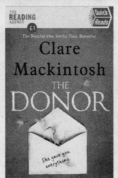

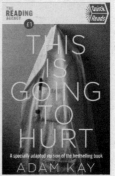

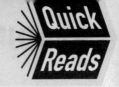

More from Quick Reads

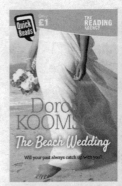

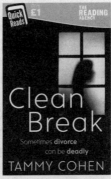

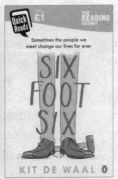

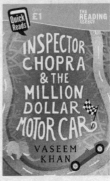

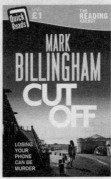

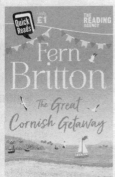

For a complete list of titles and more information
on the authors and stories visit

www.readingagency.org.uk/quickreads

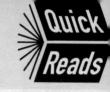
Continue your reading journey

The Reading Agency is here to help keep you
and your family reading:

Challenge yourself to complete six reads
by taking part in **Reading Ahead**
at your local library, college or workplace
readingahead.org.uk

Join **Reading Groups for Everyone** to find a
reading group and discover new books
readinggroups.org.uk

Celebrate reading on **World Book Night**
every year on 23 April
worldbooknight.org

Read with your family as part of the
Summer Reading Challenge
at your local library
summerreadingchallenge.org.uk

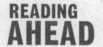

For more information, please visit our website:
readingagency.org.uk